By the same author
Mummy Laid An Egg!

RED FOX

Dr Dog.

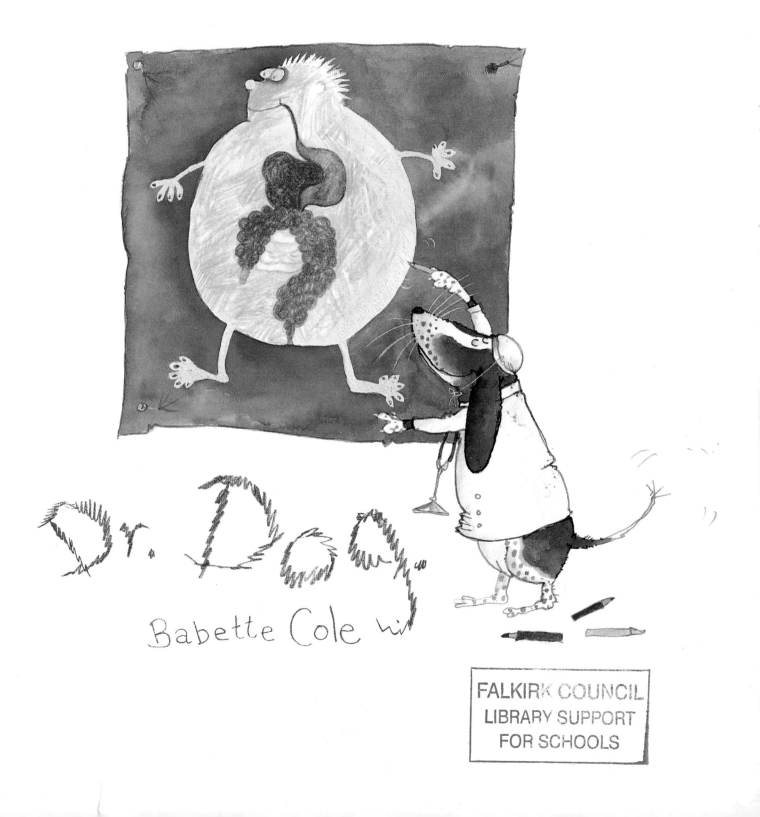

Dr. Dog

Babette Cole

This is the Gumboyle family.

And this is their dog. He is a doctor.

Dr. Dog went to
a conference in
Brazil to give a
talk about bone marrow.

While he was away Grandad and the Gumboyle children got ill.

"We'd better get him back!" said Ma Gumboyle.

So they sent a telemessage to Brazil. . .

. . . and Dr. Dog came home.

Kurt Gumboyle had been secretly smoking in the
bicycle shed. He had a wicked cough.
"It's not good to smoke,"
said Dr. Dog.

Cough!

Cough! Cough!

"These spongy things inside our chests are called lungs. They are our breathing machines.

Smoking fills them up with dirty tar. Then they don't work properly and so we cough."

Gerty Gumboyle had not been wearing
her raincoat and hat.

She caught a cold and
got a sore throat.

The germs attacked her tonsils.

"She's got tonsillitis," said Dr. Dog.

Kev Gumboyle was scratching his head like mad.

"He's got nits!" said Dr. Dog.
"These are eggs laid
by little insects
called lice.

This is one!
They live in
your hair!"

He plastered Kev's hair with smelly shampoo to kill the lice and Kev had to wear it all day at school.

"Never swap combs and brushes with anyone!" said Dr. Dog.

Ha Ha!

Ha!

Baby Gumboyle did not wash his hands
after going to the toilet.
Then he sucked
his thumb.

And he let other children
stick their fingers up
his nose.

So he got tummy ache.

"He's caught worms," said Dr. Dog.
"They are breeding in his tubes."

"The worms wriggle inside you until they reach your bottom. There they lay itchy little eggs.

If you scratch your bum, the eggs go under your fingernails."

"Sucking your thumb makes the eggs go back into your tummy, where they hatch into more worms again!

Never scratch your bum and suck your thumb!" said Dr. Dog.

WORM medicin

Fiona Gumboyle felt dizzy.

"It's all those cartwheels she's been turning!" laughed her parents.

"Rubbish," growled Dr. Dog. "She's got earache."

"There are tiny bones inside our ears that help us balance.

Earache can affect these
and make us dizzy."

Dr. Dog gave her
some pills.

Grandad had been eating too many baked beans
and drinking too much beer.

"He's got terrible wind!" said Dr. Dog.

"Here's a picture of your inside tubes.

Beer and baked beans make gases in your tummy. The only way they can escape is to blast out of your bottom!"

"It's disgusting," Dr. Dog told Ma and Pa Gumboyle. "If you don't take better care of your family,
there will be a serious accident."

"So what!" said the Gumboyles, "we've got you to look after us haven't we!"

Meanwhile Grandad's dangerous gases were building up and . . .

. . . he farted so hard he blew the roof
right off the house!

BAN

"Told you so," said Dr. Dog.

Once the roof had been put back and he had made everyone better, Dr. Dog felt ill himself.

"You're suffering from stress, Dog," said his doctor.
"What you need is a holiday away from that pesky family."

"Just what the doctor ordered," said Dr. Dog.
"They'll never find me here!"

"Oh no!" said Dr. Dog.

A Red Fox Book

Published by Random House Children's Books, 20 Vauxhall Bridge Road, London SW1V 2SA

A division of Random House UK Ltd. London Melbourne Sydney Auckland Johannesburg and agencies throughout the world

Copyright © Babette Cole 1994

1 3 5 7 9 10 8 6 4 2

First published by Jonathan Cape Limited 1994. Red Fox edition 1996

Printed in Hong Kong

RANDOM HOUSE UK Limited Reg. No. 954009

ISBN 0 09 965081 9